BLENDING WELLNESS

The Ultimate Guide to Juicing for a Healthier Life

Mary P. Corey

Introduction

Understanding Diabetes

Diabetes is an ongoing condition where the body battles to manage glucose levels. There are two fundamental sorts: Type 1, where the safe framework assaults insulin-delivering cells, and Type 2, normally connected to way of life factors. Checking glucose, a fair eating regimen and customary activity are vital for overseeing diabetes.

In Type 1 diabetes, the pancreas doesn't create insulin, requiring everyday insulin infusions. Type 2 diabetes includes insulin obstruction, where cells don't answer successfully to insulin. The two sorts can prompt entanglements like coronary illness, kidney issues, and nerve harm on the off chance that not overseen well. Way of life changes, prescription, and ordinary check-ups assume key parts in diabetes the executives.

Blood glucose checking is key in diabetes the executives. High glucose (hyperglycemia) and low glucose (hypoglycemia) can have serious outcomes. Carb counting manages feasts, and insulin changes might be essential. Confusions like diabetic retinopathy, neuropathy, and cardiovascular issues require watchful consideration. It's crucial to cultivate an all-encompassing methodology, tending to physical and close-to-home prosperity.

A decent eating routine for diabetes incorporates a blend of complicated starches, lean proteins, and solid fats. Standard active work helps with glucose control and the weight of the board. Prescriptions like oral antidiabetic medications or insulin infusions are in many cases recommended in light of individual requirements. Diabetes self-administration schooling furnishes people with the information and abilities to explore day-to-day difficulties. Standard clinical check-ups and screenings add to early discovery and anticipation of confusion. Way of life changes and a proactive methodology enable those with diabetes to have solid existences.

Notwithstanding actual well-being, diabetes the executives include observing close-to-home prosperity. Stress can affect glucose levels, so stress the executives' procedures are helpful. Support from companions, family, or care groups can give important consolation. Ceaseless progressions in innovation, such as persistent glucose observing frameworks and insulin siphons, improve accuracy in diabetes care. Research on new meds and treatments stays continuous, offering expected further developed medicines and inevitable fixes. Remaining educated, proactive, and versatile is key in exploring the powerful scene of diabetes on the board.

Normal eye assessments are essential for distinguishing and forestalling diabetic retinopathy, a typical difficulty influencing the eyes. Foot care is additionally fundamental, as diabetes can prompt neuropathy and course issues, expanding the gamble of foot issues. Smoking discontinuance is unequivocally encouraged, as it compounds diabetes-related inconveniences. Rest assumes a part as well; insufficient rest can influence glucose levels. Individualized care plans, taking into account factors like age and comorbidities, add to viable diabetes the executives. Continuously counsel medical services experts for customized guidance and changes following your diabetes care plan.

Types of Diabetes

Type 1 Diabetes: Normally analyzed in youth, it happens when the resistant framework erroneously assaults and obliterates insulin-delivering beta cells in the pancreas. Individuals with Type 1 diabetes need insulin infusions.

Type 2 Diabetes: Commonly created in grown-ups, frequently because of insulin opposition. Way of life factors like eating regimen and exercise assume a significant part. The executives incorporate way-of-life changes, oral prescriptions, and once-in-a-while insulin.

Gestational Diabetes: This happens during pregnancy when the body can't deliver sufficient insulin to meet the additional necessities. It ordinarily settles after labor, yet it builds the gamble of creating Type 2 diabetes later.

Different Sorts: There are interesting structures like monogenic diabetes and auxiliary diabetes, coming about because of explicit hereditary circumstances or other ailments, separately.

Understanding the sort is critical for appropriate administration and treatment.

Prediabetes: Before creating Type 2 diabetes, a few people experience high glucose levels however not sufficiently high for a diabetes determination. It's an admonition sign and a chance to make a way of life changes to forestall movement.

Dormant Immune System Diabetes in Grown-ups (LADA): Some of the time alluded to as "Type 1.5 diabetes," LADA imparts attributes to both Kind 1 and Type 2. It's a sluggish advancing type of immune system diabetes that frequently shows up in adulthood.

Neonatal Diabetes: This uncommon type of diabetes is created in the initial half year of life. It very well might be transient or super durable, requiring long-lasting administration.

Development Beginning Diabetes of the Youthful (MODY): An intriguing, acquired type of diabetes generally analyzed before age 25. It results from changes in unambiguous qualities influencing insulin creation.

Each type has particular attributes, and customized treatment plans are fundamental for powerful diabetes executives.

Auxiliary Diabetes: This structure results from other ailments, like infections of the pancreas, certain drugs, or hormonal problems. Treating the fundamental reason is urgent in overseeing optional diabetes.

Drug-Initiated Diabetes: A few prescriptions, similar to specific steroids or antipsychotics, can instigate diabetes as a secondary effect. Checking glucose levels and working with medical services suppliers to oversee drug-related impacts is significant.

Keep in mind, that exact conclusion and fitting administration are crucial, as various kinds of diabetes require various ways to deal with treatment and way of life changes.

2.2 Managing Blood Sugar Levels
Benefits of Juicing for Diabetes

Nutrient-Rich Ingredients

Consider integrating vegetables like kale, spinach, and cucumber for a diabetes-accommodating juice. Incorporate low-glycemic natural products like berries and green apples, and add a bit of ginger or turmeric for flavor and expected calming benefits.

incorporate celery, harsh gourd, and carrots in your diabetes-accommodating juice for added supplements. These fixings give nutrients, minerals, and cancer prevention agents while assisting with keeping up with stable glucose levels. Hold segments under control and focus on vegetables over natural products to limit sugar content.

Consider integrating spices like cilantro and mint into your diabetes-accommodating juice for added flavor without added sugars. Chia seeds or flaxseeds can likewise be helpful, giving omega-3 unsaturated fats and fiber. Explore different avenues regarding blends to track down an equilibrium that suits your taste while meeting your wholesome necessities. Keep in mind, that balance is critical, and it's crucial to screen your glucose levels routinely.

To improve the dietary profile of your diabetes-accommodating juice, add a sprinkle of lemon or lime juice for an explosion of citrus flavor without spiking glucose. Moreover, consolidating a limited quantity of avocado can contribute solid fats, advancing satiety. Continuously hold back nothing blend of fixings to guarantee a wide range of supplements. Change recipes because of individual inclinations and dietary prerequisites.

Consider remembering aloe vera juice for your diabetes-accommodating invention for its possible mitigating properties and stomach-related benefits. Moreover, cinnamon might add a touch of pleasantness without raising glucose levels essentially. Be aware of part estimates, and recollect that singular reactions to food varieties can change, so screen your body's responses to various fixings.

Integrating green tea into your diabetes-accommodating juice can offer extra cell reinforcements and potential glucose guideline benefits. Furthermore, including a limited quantity of beetroot for its normal pleasantness and potential circulatory strain bringing down properties can be valuable. Continue to explore different avenues regarding different mixes, however, consistently focus on the guidance of your medical services group to guarantee the most ideal decisions for your singular wellbeing needs.

Impact on Insulin Sensitivity

Squeezing can influence insulin awareness in people with diabetes. While new leafy food juices can give supplements, they can likewise raise glucose levels because of their normal sugars. Checking carb intake is urgent.

Squeezing might prompt a fast deluge of sugars, possibly influencing glucose levels. Counting fiber-rich fixings or matching juices with protein can assist with alleviating this impact. Nonetheless, control and individualized dietary contemplations are fundamental for those with diabetes to keep up with ideal insulin awareness.

Also, entire leafy foods offer more fiber compared with their squeezed partners. Fiber manages glucose levels and works on by and large metabolic wellbeing. Offsetting squeezing with a balanced eating routine and normal activity can add to better insulin responsiveness in people with diabetes.

It means a lot to take note of that while squeezing can be important for a sound eating regimen, depending exclusively on juices might miss the mark on an essential equilibrium of supplements. Entire food varieties give a more extensive scope of nutrients, minerals, and fiber, adding to supported energy and better generally speaking well-being. To upgrade insulin responsiveness, center around a different, supplement-rich eating regimen, and keep a way of life that incorporates customary actual work.

Consider integrating low-glycemic products of the soil into your juices, as they mildly affect glucose levels. Models incorporate salad greens, cucumber, and berries. Exploring different avenues regarding different fixing blends and piece sizes can help tweak your way of dealing with squeezing for better insulin awareness.

Integrating sound fats like avocado or nuts into your juices can likewise dial back the assimilation of sugars, possibly assisting with settling glucose levels. Also, scattering your juice utilization for the day instead of polishing off huge amounts on the double might offer better glucose control. Continuously hold back nothing diet that lines up with your particular wholesome requirements.

Recollect that singular reactions to squeezing can change, so it's significant to screen your glucose levels consistently and change your eating routine in like manner. Be aware of piece sizes, pick various vivid foods grown from the ground, and think about the general effect on your day-to-day starch consumption. Finding some kind of harmony between squeezing, entire food sources, and different parts of a sound way of life, like customary actual work, can add to better insulin responsiveness for people with diabetes.

While squeezing can offer dietary advantages, it's crucial to know about likely difficulties, like the convergence of sugars in certain juices. Pick a different scope of vegetables, consolidate lean proteins, and keep a fair eating routine to help general well-being.

Chapter 1 Essential Juicing Tools and Ingredients

Choosing the Right Juicer

For a diabetes patient, a sluggish chewing juicer is best as it holds more supplements and delivers juice with a lower glycemic record. This assists in dealing with blood sugar levels successfully. Also, centers around vegetables with lower sugar content, such as salad greens and cucumber, as opposed to high-sugar organic products.

Consider a juicer with simple cleanup to support standard use and consolidate fiber-rich fixings to slow sugar retention. Select green vegetables like kale and spinach, which are supplement thick and insignificantly affect glucose. Explore different avenues regarding low-glycemic natural products like berries. Screen segment sizes to control starch consumption, and recall that entire foods grown from the ground are many times better compared to juice for overseeing glucose.

Pick a juicer that separates squeeze effectively to boost yield and lessen squander. Search for one with flexible settings to control mash content because of individual inclination. Remember that control is critical, and it's fitting to incorporate different fixings to guarantee an even healthful profile.

Here is a diabetes-accommodating juice recipe:

Green Citrus Pleasure:

Fixings:

2 cups spinach leaves

1 cucumber

2 stems celery

1 green apple (eliminate seeds)

1/2 lemon (stripped)

1-inch ginger (discretionary for added character)

Guidelines:

Wash every one of the fixings completely.

Cut the cucumber, celery, and apple into sensible pieces.

Strip the lemon and eliminate the seeds from the apple.

Feed the fixings through your chewing juicer.

Mix the juice well to combine flavors.

Pour over ice and appreciate!

This recipe consolidates low-glycemic vegetables with a dash of regular pleasantness from the apple. Change fixings given individual taste and talk with your medical care supplier to guarantee it lines up with your dietary requirements.

Here is another diabetes-accommodating juice recipe:

Berry Happiness Boost:

Fixings:

1 cup blueberries

1 cup raspberries

1 cup kale leaves

1 cucumber

1/2 lime (stripped)

1 tablespoon chia seeds (discretionary, for added fiber)

Guidelines:

Wash every one of the berries, kale, and cucumber completely.

Cut the cucumber into sensible pieces.

Feed the blueberries, raspberries, kale, cucumber, and striped lime through your juicer.

In the case of utilizing chia seeds, mix them into the juice after squeezing.

Pour over ice and partake in the reviving berry goodness!

This recipe joins the cell reinforcements from berries with the nourishing advantages of kale, while the cucumber adds a hydrating component. Change amounts to suit your taste inclinations and counsel your medical services supplier for customized exhortation.

Diabetes–Friendly Fruits and Vegetables

Diabetics can pick low-glycemic natural products like berries, cherries, and apples. Non-boring vegetables like mixed greens, broccoli, and cauliflower are additionally great decisions.

Other diabetes-accommodating organic products incorporate peaches, plums, and pears. Concerning vegetables, pick choices like chime peppers, zucchini, and spinach. These decisions can assist with overseeing glucose levels. Keep in mind that control and equilibrium are vital.

Incorporate avocados for sound fats and fiber. Berries like strawberries and blueberries are wealthy in cancer prevention agents. Pick cruciferous vegetables, for example, Brussels fledglings and cabbage. Try different things with an assortment to guarantee a balanced, nutritious eating routine while overseeing diabetes.

Integrate citrus natural products like oranges and grapefruits for L-ascorbic acid. Tomatoes, despite being natural products, are low in carbs and can be essential for a diabetes-accommodating eating regimen. Also, pick beautiful vegetables like carrots and peppers for added supplements. Focus on entire, natural food sources for ideal well-being.

Consider adding kiwi for its fiber and vitamin K substance. Green beans and asparagus are great vegetable decisions because of their low effect on glucose. Investigate different choices to keep a decent eating routine that lines up with diabetes the executive's rules.

Incorporate melons like melon and watermelon with some restraint, as they have generally lower glycemic records. Mixed greens, for example, kale and Swiss chard are fantastic decisions for their wholesome thickness. Make sure to zero in on segment control and screen your glucose levels routinely for ideal administration.

Increases like cucumber and radishes are low-carb and can improve plates of mixed greens or tidbits. Pick natural products like guava and apricots, which give fiber and nutrients. Go for the gold offset diet with a blend of varieties and supplements while being aware of your singular dietary necessities.

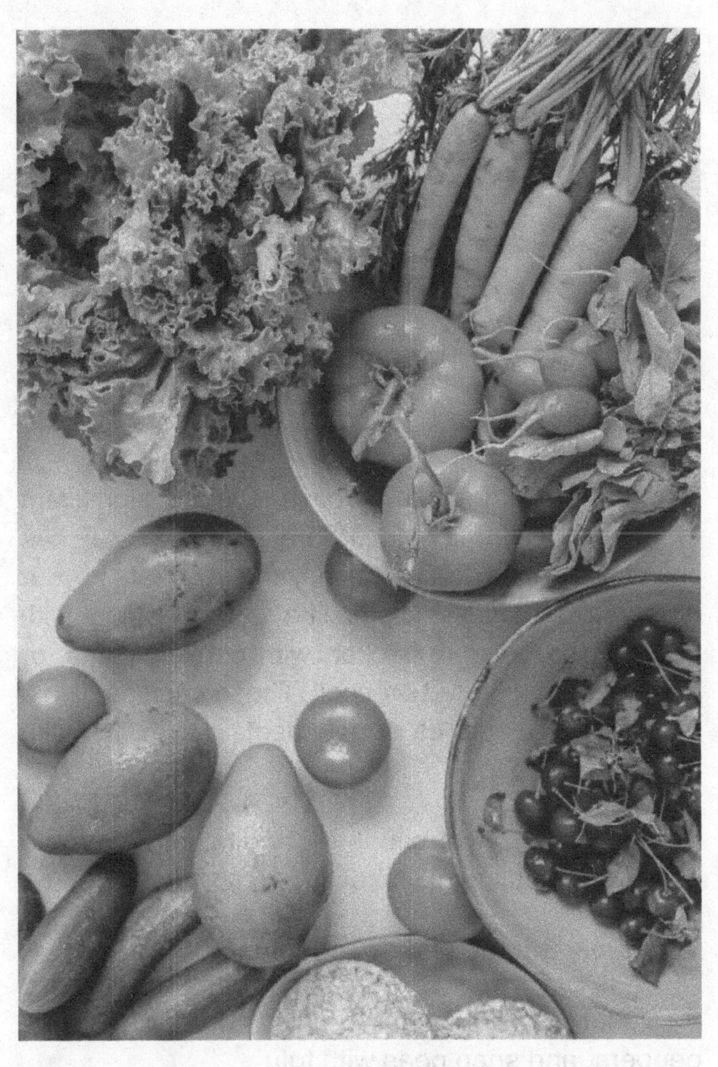

Chapter 2: Creating Balanced and Low–Glycemic Juices

Recipes for Stable Blood Sugar

Keeping up with stable glucose levels is significant for general well-being. Incorporate complex starches like entire grains, lean proteins, and solid fats in your dinners. Consider recipes like quinoa salad with veggies, barbecued chicken with cooked yams, or salmon with steamed broccoli. These choices give a reasonable blend of supplements to assist with directing glucose.

The following are a couple of additional recipes to assist with settling glucose:

Vegetable Sautéed food with Tofu:

Pan-sear vivid vegetables like broccoli, chime peppers, and snap peas with tofu.

Utilize a low-sugar, soy-based sauce for some zing.

Serve over cauliflower rice for a low-carb choice.

Chickpea and Spinach Curry:

Join chickpeas, spinach, and tomatoes in a curry sauce with flavors like turmeric and cumin.

Present with quinoa or earthy-colored rice for fiber support.

Barbecued Turkey and Veggie Sticks:

String lean turkey 3D squares, cherry tomatoes, zucchini, and mushrooms onto sticks.

Barbecue until the turkey is cooked and the veggies are delicate.

Mediterranean Plate of Mixed Greens with Barbecued Chicken:

Throw together blended greens, cherry tomatoes, cucumber, olives, and feta.

Top with barbecued chicken and dress with olive oil and lemon.

Broiler Prepared Fish with Asparagus:

Put fish filets on a baking sheet, and encompass them with asparagus lances.

Season with spices, lemon, and a shower of olive oil before baking.

Keep in mind, that segment control is vital, and it's fitting to screen your glucose levels consistently. Change recipes given your dietary inclinations.

The following are a couple of additional recipes with an emphasis on settling glucose:

Lentil and Vegetable Soup:

Consolidate lentils, carrots, celery, and spinach in a stock-based soup.

Add spices like thyme and rosemary for some extra zing.

Prepared Yam Fries:

Cut yams into fries, throw with olive oil, and prepare until fresh.

Present with a side of Greek yogurt for plunging.

Salmon and Quinoa Bowl:

Barbecue or prepare salmon and serve over a bed of cooked quinoa.

Add cooked vegetables like Brussels fledglings and sprinkle with lemon.

Egg and Vegetable Omelet:

Whisk eggs and cook with various vivid veggies like ringer peppers, tomatoes, and spinach.

Top with avocado cuts for solid fats.

Cauliflower Broiled Rice with Shrimp:

Beat cauliflower in a food processor to make rice-sized pieces.

Pan-sear with shrimp, blended vegetables, and a low-sodium soy sauce.

Greek Yogurt Parfait:

Layer Greek yogurt with new berries, a sprinkle of nuts, and a shower of honey for pleasantness.

These recipes integrate supplement thick fixings to help glucose dependability. Make sure to fit these ideas to your particular dietary requirements.

The following are a couple of extra recipes:

Turkey and Vegetable Skillet:

Earthy-colored lean ground turkey in a skillet with diced chime peppers, onions, and spinach.

Season with spices like oregano and basil.

Chia Seed Pudding:

Blend chia seeds with unsweetened almond milk, and let it sit for the time being.

Top with new berries and a sprinkle of nuts.

Stuffed Chime Peppers with Quinoa and Dark Beans:

Cook a combination of quinoa, dark beans, corn, and flavors.

Stuff chime peppers with the combination and heat until delicate.

Chicken and Broccoli Pan fried food:

Pan-sear chicken tenders with broccoli, snow peas, and water chestnuts.

Utilize a light teriyaki sauce for some extra zing.

Avocado and Fish Salad:

Join canned fish with diced avocado, cherry tomatoes, and cucumber.

Dress with olive oil and lemon juice.

Spaghetti Squash with Turkey Bolognese:

Broil spaghetti squash and top with a lean turkey Bolognese sauce.

Sprinkle with ground Parmesan for added character.

These recipes center around integrating entire, natural food varieties that can add to stable glucose levels. Change fixings because of your inclinations and dietary necessities.

The following are a couple of additional recipes that focus on stable glucose:

Cabbage and Turkey Sautéed food:

Saute ground turkey with destroyed cabbage, carrots, and snow peas.

Season with ginger, garlic, and low-sodium soy sauce.

Bean and Vegetable Burrito Bowl:

Blend dark beans in with broiled vegetables like chime peppers, onions, and corn.

Serve over a bed of earthy-colored rice or cauliflower rice.

Spinach and Feta Stuffed Chicken Bosom:

Stuff chicken bosoms with a combination of sautéed spinach and feta cheddar.

Heat until chicken is cooked through.

Cauliflower and Chickpea Curry:

Stew cauliflower florets and chickpeas in a curry sauce made with tomatoes and coconut milk.

Serve over quinoa.

Eggplant and Mozzarella Prepare:

Layer cut eggplant with pureed tomatoes and part-skim mozzarella.

Heat until effervescent and brilliant.

Green Smoothie Bowl:

Mix spinach, kale, banana, and almond milk.

Top with chia seeds, cut almonds, and new berries.

Make sure to screen segment measures and pick entire, supplement-thick food sources to assist with keeping up with stable glucose levels. Adjust these recipes to suit your taste inclinations and dietary prerequisites

Portion Control and Timing

For diabetes, center around offset dinners with controlled segments, divided over the day. Hold back nothing admission.

Partition your everyday admission into more modest, regular dinners to assist with settling glucose levels. Select entire grains, lean proteins, and a lot of vegetables. Screen your glucose consistently to comprehend what various food sources and timings mean for your levels.

Incorporate high-fiber food sources to dial back processing and ingestion of carbs, managing glucose. Pick sound fats, like avocados or nuts, and remain hydrated. Customary active work can likewise add to more readily glucose control.

Consider integrating food sources with a low glycemic record (GI), as they smallerly affect glucose levels. Be aware of sweet refreshments and breaking-point liquor admission. Foster an everyday practice for dinners and snacks to keep up with consistency. Change segment sizes in light of your movement level and any progressions in the prescription.

Explore different avenues regarding careful eating, focusing on appetite and totality signals. Investigate cooking techniques like steaming, barbecuing, or baking as opposed to broiling. Incorporate different bright vegetables to guarantee a wide scope of supplements. Keep a food journal to follow feasts, distinguish examples, and make informed changes. Go for the gold-adjusted, practical way to deal with sustenance.

Consolidate pressure on the board methods, as stress can affect glucose levels. Rest is likewise significant; hold back nothing rest timetable to help by and large prosperity. Routinely check your glucose levels and note any examples to refine your methodology.

Chapter 3: Incorporating Superfoods

Berries, Leafy Greens, and More

Berries like blueberries and strawberries are wealthy in cancer prevention agents. Salad greens, for example, spinach and kale give fundamental supplements. Other superfoods incorporate chia seeds for omega-3 unsaturated fats and yams for nutrients. Integrating an assortment of these into your eating routine can help your general well-being.

Incorporate quinoa for protein and fiber, nuts like almonds for sound fats, and turmeric known for its mitigating properties. Salmon is an incredible wellspring of omega-3s, while Greek yogurt offers probiotics. Different superfoods make a balanced and nutritious eating regimen.

Add dull chocolate for cell reinforcements, avocados for solid fats, and broccoli for nutrients. Lentils give protein and iron, and green tea offers cancer prevention agents. Joining these superfoods upholds generally speaking prosperity and can add to a fair eating routine.

Consider consolidating acai berries for cancer prevention agents, hemp seeds for omega-3s, and ginger for mitigating benefits. Furthermore, garlic has safe helping properties, and beets are plentiful in nutrients and minerals. Exploring different avenues regarding these superfoods enhances your feast.

the following are two superfood-rich recipes:

Quinoa Salad with Berries and Greens:

Cooked quinoa

Blended berries (blueberries, strawberries)

Cleaved spinach and kale

Feta cheddar

Balsamic vinaigrette dressing

Prepare all fixings together for a reviving and supplement stuffed salad.

Salmon and Avocado Sushi Bowl:

Cooked quinoa or earthy colored rice

Barbecued salmon

Cut avocado

Ocean growth strips

Soy sauce or tamari

Sesame seeds

Organize these fixings in a bowl for a dismantled sushi experience with a portion of omega-3s and sound fats.

Partake in these superfood-stuffed dinners!

Here is another superfood-rich recipe:

Yam and Chickpea Buddha Bowl:

Cooked yam pieces

Cooked quinoa

Chickpeas (cooked or sautéed)

Cut avocado

Kale or spinach (rubbed with olive oil)

Tahini dressing

Join these components in a bowl for a feeding and delightful Buddha Bowl that gives an equilibrium of fiber, protein, and fundamental supplements.

Boosting Antioxidants and Anti-Inflammatory Properties

To help cell reinforcements and mitigating properties, consider consolidating superfoods like berries, salad greens, nuts, and seeds into your eating regimen. These food sources are plentiful in nutrients, minerals, and phytochemicals that advance by and large well-being. Furthermore, flavors like turmeric and ginger have powerful calming impacts. Make sure to keep a decent and different eating regimen for ideal advantages.

Incorporate food sources like dim chocolate, green tea, and greasy fish (like salmon) for added cell reinforcements and omega-3 unsaturated fats. Underline a brilliant exhibit of leafy foods to expand the supplement assortment. Explore different avenues regarding spices like rosemary and oregano, known for their cell reinforcement properties. Remain hydrated with water and natural teas, supporting general prosperity. Ordinary activity supplements these endeavors, adding to mitigating impacts.

Investigate consolidating food sources like chia seeds, flaxseeds, and pecans for omega-3 unsaturated fats. Quinoa and yams offer assorted supplements and mitigating benefits. Consider adding aged food varieties like yogurt or kimchi to help stomach well-being, impacting aggravation. Brighten up feasts with garlic and onions, known for their resistant helping and calming properties. Take a stab at a balanced eating routine, zeroing in on entire, natural food sources to outfit the most extreme medical advantages.

Try not to neglect the force of green vegetables like kale and spinach, high in cell reinforcements and mitigating compounds. Citrus organic products give a L-ascorbic acid lift, upgrading safe capability. Turmeric, with its dynamic compound curcumin, is an intense mitigating zest. Olive oil, rich in monounsaturated fats and cell reinforcements, can be a solid decision for cooking. Consistency in consolidating these superfoods into your eating routine is critical to receiving long-haul well-being rewards.

Here is a basic and nutritious recipe:

Quinoa Salad with Berries and Spinach:

Fixings:

1 cup quinoa (cooked by bundle directions)

2 cups new spinach leaves

1 cup blended berries (blueberries, strawberries, raspberries)

1/4 cup feta cheddar, disintegrated

1/4 cup pecans, hacked

2 tablespoons balsamic vinaigrette

Salt and pepper to taste

Directions:

Cook quinoa and let it cool.

In a huge bowl, join quinoa, new spinach, blended berries, disintegrated feta, and slashed pecans.

Shower balsamic vinaigrette over the serving of mixed greens and throw delicately to join.

Season with salt and pepper to taste.

Serve chilled and partake in a delightful, cell reinforcement-rich dish!

Go ahead and tweak the recipe by adding your most loved superfoods or changing the amounts because of your inclinations.

Here is a recipe for a scrumptious and mitigating smoothie:

Turmeric Mango Smoothie:

Fixings:

1 cup frozen mango pieces

1/2 banana

1/2 teaspoon turmeric powder (or ground new turmeric)

1/2 teaspoon ginger (new or ground)

1 tablespoon chia seeds

1 cup coconut water or almond milk

Ice 3D squares (discretionary)

Directions:

In a blender, consolidate frozen mango pieces, banana, turmeric powder, ginger, and chia seeds.

Pour in coconut water or almond milk for a smooth consistency.

Add ice solid shapes whenever wanted and mix until smooth.

Fill a glass and partake in this reviving and mitigating smoothie.

This smoothie joins the tropical pleasantness of mango with the mitigating advantages of turmeric and ginger, making it a scrumptious and well-being-helping treat.

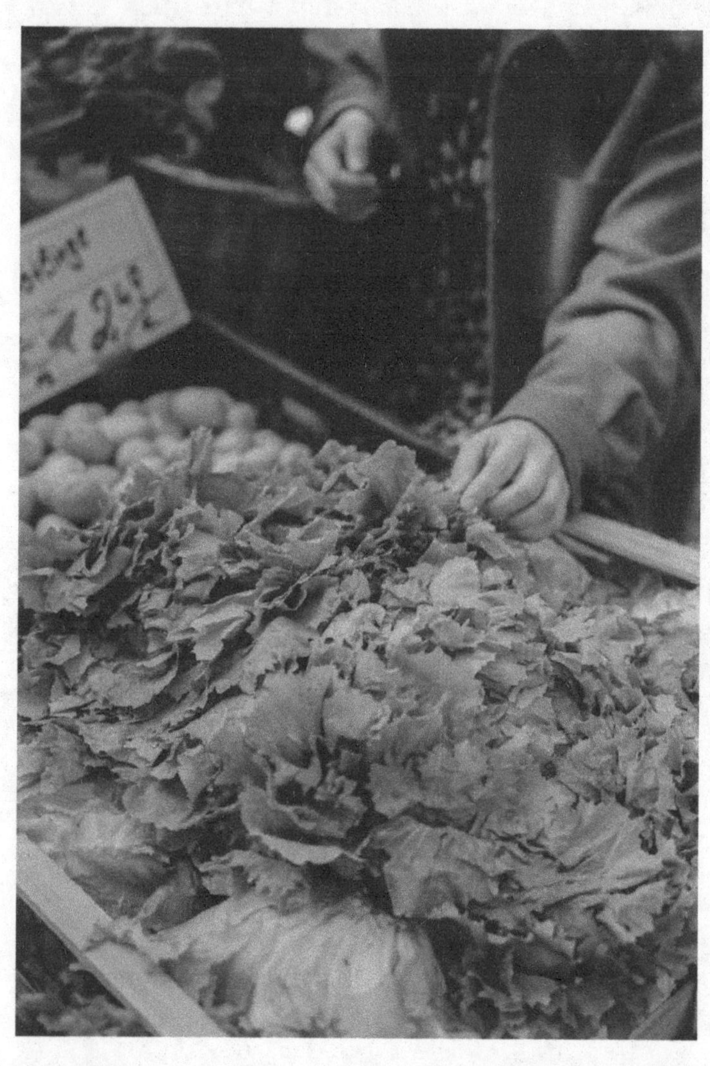

This smoothie joins the top abundances of
changes in the natural advantages of humans
and plants, including a scrumptuous and exuberant
shaping force.

Chapter 4: Creating Balanced and Low-Glycemic Juices

Recipes for Stable Blood Sugar

To keep up with stable glucose levels, center around a reasonable eating regimen with entire food varieties. Incorporate lean proteins, high-fiber vegetables, and complex carbs. For a low-glycemic juice, take a stab at mixing spinach, cucumber, and berries for a supplement-rich choice. Make sure to screen segment estimates and pick entire natural products over natural product juices.

Here is an example day of feasts for stable glucose:

Breakfast:

Cereal with cut almonds and new berries.

Fried eggs with spinach.

Green tea or dark espresso.

Early in the day Tidbit:

Greek yogurt with chia seeds.

A little apple or pear.

Lunch:

Barbecued chicken or tofu salad with blended greens and brilliant veggies.

Quinoa or earthy-colored rice as a side.

Water with lemon or homegrown tea.

Evening Bite:

Carrot and cucumber sticks with hummus.

Modest bunch of nuts (almonds, pecans, or pistachios).

Supper:

Heated or barbecued salmon with cooked Brussels sprouts.

Steamed broccoli or asparagus.

Yam or cauliflower squash.

Low-Glycemic Juice:

Spinach, cucumber, and a portion of a cup of blended berries (blueberries, raspberries).

Mix with water or coconut water for hydration.

Keep in mind, that spreading dinners equally for the day and screening your starch intake is fundamental. This example plan gives an equilibrium between supplements and keeps up with consistent glucose levels.

here are extra tips and contemplations for keeping up with stable glucose:

Hydration:

Drink a lot of water over the day to remain hydrated.

Natural teas, similar to chamomile or green tea, can be great decisions.

Nibbling:

Choose snacks with protein and fiber to assist with controlling cravings and glucose.

Models incorporate cut ringer peppers with guacamole or a small bunch of cherry tomatoes with mozzarella.

Solid Fats:

Incorporate wellsprings of solid fats, like avocados, olive oil, and nuts, in your dinners to advance satiety.

Entire Grains:

Pick entire grains like quinoa, grain, and entire wheat over refined grains for supported energy.

Feast Timing:

Hold back nothing timings to assist with controlling glucose.

Stay away from delayed periods without eating; consider having more modest, adjusted snacks if necessary.

Segment Control:

Be aware of part sizes to forestall indulging and assist with keeping up with stable glucose levels.

Active work:

Standard activity is pivotal for the glucose of the executives. Incorporate both vigorous and strength-preparing practices in your daily schedule.

Limit Handled Food varieties:

Limit handled and sweet food sources, as they can cause quick spikes and crashes in glucose levels.

here are some extra low-glycemic food choices and recipe thoughts:

Low-Glycemic Vegetables:

Broccoli, cauliflower, kale, zucchini, and ringer peppers are astounding decisions.

Attempt simmered Brussels sprouts with a shower of olive oil and a sprinkle of garlic for a tasty side dish.

Lean Protein Sources:

Skinless chicken bosom, turkey, tofu, and fish (like cod or halibut) are low in sugars.

Barbecue or heat chicken with spices and flavors for a delectable, protein-rich feast.

Solid Nibble Thoughts:

Curds with cherry tomatoes.

Cut cucumber with smoked salmon.

Edamame with a hint of ocean salt.

Entire Grains Choices:

Grain or bulgur can be utilized in plates of mixed greens for added surface and fiber.

Make sautéed food with quinoa rather than white rice.

Dessert Choices:

Berries with a spot of Greek yogurt.

Dim chocolate (with some restraint) for a sweet treat.

Adjusted Smoothie:

Mix spinach, cucumber, avocado, and a little piece of berries with unsweetened almond milk for a low-glycemic, supplement-pressed smoothie.

Keep in mind, that assortment is vital, and integrating a great many supplement thick food varieties into your eating regimen guarantees you get a decent blend of fundamental supplements. Explore different avenues regarding flavors and recipes to find what turns out best for your taste inclinations and glucose the executives.

here are more recipe thoughts to assist with keeping up with stable glucose levels:

Stuffed Ringer Peppers:

Fill chime peppers with a blend of lean ground turkey, dark beans, quinoa, and diced tomatoes. Prepare until the peppers are delicate.

Egg and Vegetable Wrap:

Scramble eggs with spinach, tomatoes, and mushrooms. Enclose the combination with an entire grain tortilla for a wonderful and low-glycemic breakfast or lunch.

Cauliflower Rice Bowl:

Supplant customary rice with cauliflower rice and top it with barbecued chicken or tofu, sautéed vegetables, and a shower of olive oil.

Salmon Serving of mixed greens:

Barbecued or heated salmon on a bed of leafy greens, cherry tomatoes, and cucumber cuts. Dress with a vinaigrette made with olive oil and lemon.

Lentil Soup:

Cook a good lentil soup with vegetables like carrots, celery, and spinach. Lentils are a decent wellspring of protein and fiber.

Chia Seed Pudding:

Blend chia seeds with unsweetened almond milk and allow it to sit for the time being. Top with berries and a sprinkle of nuts for a tasty and low-glycemic sweet or tidbit.

Cabbage and Turkey Pan fried food:

Pan-sear ground turkey with destroyed cabbage, broccoli, and snow peas. Season with ginger, garlic, and low-sodium soy sauce.

Spaghetti Squash with Meat Sauce:

Broil spaghetti squash and top it with natively constructed pureed tomatoes made with lean ground hamburger or turkey.

Make sure to fit these recipes as you would prefer inclinations and dietary requirements. Change segment sizes in light of your singular prerequisites, and go ahead and try different things with various spices and flavors to upgrade flavors.

Green Citrus Delight

Green Citrus Joy can be a decent, low-glycemic choice. Consolidate mixed greens, citrus natural products, and perhaps a wellspring of solid fat or protein to upgrade satiety and balance out glucose levels.

Consider a plate of mixed greens with salad greens like spinach or kale, matched with citrus natural products like oranges or grapefruits. Add some avocado or nuts for sound fats and maybe barbecued chicken for protein, making a fantastic and low-glycemic feast.

Try different things with a hand-crafted vinaigrette involving olive oil and citrus juices for added flavor without spiking glycemic levels. Make sure to zero in on entire, natural fixings to keep up with the dietary respectability of your Green Citrus Enjoyment.

Integrating fiber-rich vegetables like broccoli or chime peppers can additionally upgrade the nourishing profile and add to a slower glucose discharge. Be aware of piece measures and partake in your Green Citrus Joy as a component of a balanced, adjusted diet.

Consider including quinoa as a base for your Green Citrus Joy. Quinoa is a low-glycemic grain that adds protein and extra fiber to your feast, advancing a supported arrival of energy. Tweaking your recipe to suit individual inclinations guarantees a heavenly and adjusted dish.

To keep up with the low-glycemic nature, decide on a moderate dressing utilizing olive oil, lemon or lime juice, and spices for some extra zing. This holds added sugars within proper limits while upgrading the general taste of your Green Citrus Joy. Keep in mind that, assortment in your fixings adds to a balanced and nutritious dish.

Consider integrating spices like cilantro or mint into your Green Citrus Joy for added newness and flavor. These spices raise the taste as well as carry extra supplements and cell reinforcements to the blend, adding to the general medical advantages of your dinner.

Here is a straightforward recipe for a Green Citrus Enjoyment Salad:

Fixings:

2 cups new spinach or kale

1 cup blended greens

1 orange, stripped and portioned

1/2 avocado, diced

1/4 cup nuts (pecans or almonds)

1/2 cup cooked quinoa

Barbecued chicken bosom (discretionary)

New spices (cilantro or mint)

Dressing:

2 tablespoons olive oil

Juice of 1 lemon or lime

Salt and pepper to taste

Directions:

In a huge bowl, consolidate spinach, blended greens, orange fragments, diced avocado, nuts, and cooked quinoa.

Whenever wanted, add barbecued chicken for protein.

In a little bowl, whisk together olive oil, lemon or lime squeeze, salt, and pepper to make the dressing.

Sprinkle the dressing over the plate of mixed greens and throw tenderly to equitably cover all fixings.

Embellish with new spices like cilantro or mint.

Serve right away and partake in your Green Citrus Joy Salad!

Go ahead and alter the recipe given your inclinations and dietary requirements.

Here is one more recipe variety for a Green Citrus Enjoyment Smoothie:

Fixings:

1 cup spinach leaves

1/2 cucumber, stripped and cut

1/2 avocado

1/2 cup green grapes

Juice of 1 lime

1/2 cup coconut water or water

Ice 3D squares (discretionary)

Directions:

Place spinach, cucumber, avocado, green grapes, lime juice, and coconut water (or water) in a blender.

Whenever wanted, add ice 3D shapes for a colder surface.

Mix until smooth and rich.

Fill a glass and partake in your reviving Green Citrus Enjoyment Smoothie!

This smoothie is loaded with supplements from greens, avocado, and citrus, giving an invigorating and low-glycemic choice. Change amounts given your taste inclinations.

Berry Bliss Antioxidant Blend

Berry Ecstasy Cell Reinforcement Mix is an available blend of berries rich in cancer prevention agents, giving potential medical advantages. Blueberries, raspberries, and acai berries are normal parts known for their cancer-prevention agent properties.

This mix could offer safe help, further develop heart well-being, and add to general prosperity because of the great degrees of nutrients, minerals, and cancer-prevention agents present in berries. Consider integrating it into smoothies or as a garnish for yogurt.

Berries in this mix ordinarily contain anthocyanins, flavonoids, and L-ascorbic acid, which can assist with combating oxidative pressure, decreasing aggravation, and backing skin well-being.

Customary utilization might add to a different supplement consumption for ideal well-being.

Moreover, the fiber content in these berries might help assimilation and advance stomach well-being. The blend of different cell reinforcements could make synergistic impacts, possibly offering a more extensive scope of medical advantages past individual berry utilization.

In addition, the anthocyanins in berries have been connected to mental advantages, conceivably supporting mind well-being and lessening the gamble old enough related mental deterioration. Counting Berry Happiness Cell reinforcement Mix in your eating regimen could be a delightful method for helping your by and large wholesome profile.

Here is a straightforward recipe to make an invigorating Berry Ecstasy Cell reinforcement Smoothie:

Fixings:

1 cup Berry Rapture Cell reinforcement Mix (frozen or new)

1 banana

1/2 cup Greek yogurt

1/2 cup almond milk (or any milk of your decision)

1 tablespoon honey (discretionary for pleasantness)

Directions:

Consolidate the Berry Ecstasy Cell reinforcement Mix, banana, Greek yogurt, and almond milk in a blender.

Mix until smooth and velvety.

Taste and add honey if you lean toward a better flavor.

Fill a glass and partake in your supplement-pressed, tasty smoothie!

Go ahead and modify by adding protein powder, chia seeds, or spinach for an extra wholesome lift.

Here is a recipe for a basic Berry Joy Cell reinforcement Salad:

Fixings:

2 cups blended greens (spinach, arugula, or your decision)

1 cup Berry Ecstasy Cancer prevention agent Mix

1/2 cup feta cheddar, disintegrated

1/4 cup cleaved pecans or almonds

Balsamic vinaigrette dressing

Directions:

In a huge bowl, consolidate the blended greens, Berry Ecstasy Cell reinforcement Mix, feta cheddar, and nuts.

Sprinkle balsamic vinaigrette dressing over a plate of mixed greens.

Throw the fixings delicately until all around are joined.

Serve right away and partake in a delightful and nutritious plate of mixed greens!

Go ahead and add barbecued chicken or your protein of decision to make it a more significant feast.

Cucumber Mint Cooler

Cucumber Mint Cooler is an invigorating beverage made by mixing cucumbers, mint, lime, and here and there sugars like honey or sugar. It's ideally suited for remaining hydrated and chilling off on a hot day.

To make a Cucumber Mint Cooler, combine stripped and cut cucumbers, new mint leaves, lime squeeze, and ice in a blender. Mix until smooth, then strain the combination. You can improve it with honey or sugar whenever wanted. Serve chilled, and decorate with cucumber cuts or mint leaves for an additional touch.

Try different things with varieties by adding a sprinkle of shining water or a club soft drink to give it a bubbly turn. Change the pleasantness and sharpness levels to suit your taste inclinations. It's a flexible beverage that you can redo with various spices or even a touch of ginger for added intricacy. Partake in this reviving drink as a wonderful backup to your feasts or as an independent boost.

For an additional cooling impact, freeze cucumber cuts or mint leaves into ice shapes and use them in your Cucumber Mint Cooler. This upgrades the visual allure as well as guarantees your beverage stays chilled without weakening. Go ahead and get imaginative with the show and trimmings, maybe adding a lime wheel or a twig of mint on the edge of the glass for a final detail. Cheers to an invigorating natively constructed refreshment!

Consider matching your Cucumber Mint Cooler with light and new dishes like plates of mixed greens or barbecued vegetables. The fresh and natural notes of the beverage supplement different flavors. Moreover, you can make a bigger clump and serve it at social events or picnics — being a group pleaser is certain. Make sure to change the fixings because of your taste inclinations, as the excellence of this cooler lies in its flexibility.

To make a Cucumber Mint Cooler, you'll require:

2 medium-sized cucumbers (stripped and cut)

A modest bunch of new mint leaves

Juice of 2 limes

2-3 tablespoons of honey or sugar (conform to taste)

Ice 3D shapes

Discretionary: Shining water or club soft drink for effervescence

Go ahead and modify the amounts because of your inclinations, and remember to explore different avenues regarding the pleasantness and sharpness levels until you accomplish the ideal equilibrium for your taste buds.

Here is a basic recipe for a Cucumber Mint Cooler:

Fixings:

2 medium-sized cucumbers (stripped and cut)

A modest bunch of new mint leaves

Juice of 2 limes

2-3 tablespoons of honey or sugar (conform to taste)

Ice 3D squares

Discretionary: Shining water or club soft drink for effervescence

Directions:

In a blender, consolidate cut cucumbers, new mint leaves, lime squeeze, and honey or sugar.

Mix until smooth. On the off chance that you favor a smoother surface, you can strain the combination to eliminate mash.

Taste the blend and change pleasantness or acridity depending on the situation.

Fill glasses with ice 3D shapes.

Pour the cucumber-mint mix over the ice.

Alternatively, finish off with shining water or a club soft drink for a bubbly kick.

Mix tenderly and embellish with cucumber cuts or mint leaves.

Serve chilled and partake in your custom-made Cucumber Mint Cooler!

Go ahead and get inventive and adjust the recipe however you would prefer. Good wishes!

Here is a variety of the Cucumber Mint Cooler with a sprinkle of citrus:

Citrus Cucumber Mint Cooler:

Fixings:

2 medium-sized cucumbers (stripped and cut)

A small bunch of new mint leaves

Juice of 2 limes

Juice of 1 lemon

2-3 tablespoons of honey or sugar (change per taste)

Ice 3D squares

Discretionary: Shining water or club soft drink for effervescence

Guidelines:

Mix cut cucumbers, new mint leaves, lime juice, lemon squeeze, and honey or sugar until smooth.

Strain the blend on the off chance that you lean toward a smoother surface.

Taste and change pleasantness or corrosiveness on a case-by-case basis.

Fill glasses with ice 3D shapes.

Pour the citrus-mixed cucumber mix over the ice.

Alternatively, finish off with shining water or a club soft drink for fizz.

Mix tenderly, and embellish with citrus cuts or mint leaves.

Serve chilled and relish the invigorating Citrus Cucumber Mint Cooler!

Go ahead and tweak the recipe because of your taste inclinations. Appreciate!

Spiced Apple Pie Elixir

Flavored fruity dessert solution is in many cases a warm drink made by imbuing apple juice with flavors like cinnamon, cloves, and nutmeg. It's a comfortable and delightful beverage, ideal for fall or winter. A few varieties might incorporate fixings like ginger or vanilla for added profundity of flavor.

To make a flavored fruity dessert mixture, you can begin by warming apple juice in the oven. Add cinnamon sticks, entire cloves, and a touch of nutmeg. You can likewise incorporate a cut of new ginger or a sprinkle of vanilla concentrate for additional character.

Allow the blend to stew for around 15-20 minutes to permit the flavors to implant into the juice. Be mindful so as not to bubble it; a delicate stew is adequate. A short time later, strain the fluid to eliminate the flavors.

Serve your flavored fruity dessert remedy warm, alternatively embellishing with a cinnamon stick or a cut of apple. It's a great and consoling beverage, ideal for crisp days. Appreciate!

If you're feeling bold, you can alter your flavored fruity dessert solution further. The following are a couple of thoughts:

Citrus Curve: Add a sprinkle of citrus by pressing in some new orange or lemon juice. It adds a fiery and splendid component to the warm remedy.

Maple Pleasantness: Upgrade the pleasantness with a dash of maple syrup. Change as indicated by your taste inclinations to adjust the flavors.

Whipped Cream Beating: For a debauched touch, top your flavored fruity dessert remedy with a dab of whipped cream. Sprinkle a touch of cinnamon on top for an additional treat.

Boozy Choice: For an adult variant, consider adding a sprinkle of whiskey or dim rum. It makes a warm and consoling grown-up refreshment.

Go ahead and trial and design the remedy to suit your taste inclinations. Partake in the comfortable kinds of flavored fruity dessert!

The following are a couple more imaginative turns for your flavored fruity dessert solution:

Chai Combination: Mix the apple juice with chai tea packs or free chai flavors. This mix of customary fruity dessert flavors and chai adds intricacy and profundity to the solution.

Caramel Sprinkle: Improve things by showering a touch of caramel sauce into your flavored fruity dessert remedy. A great expansion supplements the apple flavor.

Keep in mind that the magnificence of this remedy is its flexibility, so make sure to use various fixings until you find the ideal mix for your taste buds. Partake in your altered flavored fruity dessert solution!

The following are a couple more innovative turns for your flavored fruity dessert mixture:

Homegrown Concordance: Implant your solution with natural components like new rosemary or thyme. These spices can add a remarkable and fragrant contort, carrying an exquisite note to the sweet fruity dessert flavor.

Coconut Comfortable: For a tropical touch, add a sprinkle of coconut milk or coconut cream to your flavored fruity dessert remedy. The mix of warm flavors and coconut makes a soothing and colorful mix.

Go ahead and join these ideas or imagine your varieties. The excellence of this mixture is its versatility to suit various preferences. Partake in your imaginative mixtures!

how about we keep the inventiveness streaming:

Berry Euphoria: Present an explosion of fruity goodness by adding a small bunch of new berries like raspberries or blackberries to your flavored fruity dessert remedy. The poignancy of the berries can supplement the pleasantness of the juice.

Pumpkin Zest Combination: Embrace the fall seasons significantly more by consolidating a touch of pumpkin flavor. You can either utilize a pre-made pumpkin zest mix or make your own with a blend of cinnamon, nutmeg, ginger, and cloves.

Tea Mixture: Supplant some or all of the apple juice with a delightful tea, like dark tea or a natural mix. The tea adds intricacy, and you can explore different avenues regarding different tea assortments to track down your favored mix.

Go ahead and blend and match these ideas to make a flavored fruity dessert remedy that suits your taste buds impeccably. Partake in the wonderful excursion of making extraordinary and comfortable refreshments!

Here is a straightforward recipe for a Flavored Fruity dessert Remedy:

Fixings:

4 cups apple juice

2 cinnamon sticks

5 entire cloves

1/4 teaspoon ground nutmeg

Discretionary: 1 cut of new ginger or 1/2 teaspoon of vanilla concentrate

Guidelines:

In a pan, join the apple juice, cinnamon sticks, entire cloves, and ground nutmeg.

If you're utilizing new ginger or vanilla concentrate, add it to the combination.

Heat the combination over medium intensity until it starts to stew. Be careful not to heat it to the point of boiling; a delicate stew is adequate.

Allow it to stew for 15-20 minutes to permit the flavors to imbue into the juice.

Eliminate the pot from intensity and strain the fluid to eliminate the flavors.

Serve the flavored fruity dessert mixture warm. Alternatively, decorate with a cinnamon stick or a cut of apple.

Go ahead and tweak the recipe by integrating a portion of the inventive turns referenced before. Partake in your flavorful and consoling Flavored Fruity dessert Solution!

Here is a variety of the Flavored Fruity dessert Solution with a citrus curve:

Citrus-Injected Flavored Fruity Dessert Remedy:

Fixings:

4 cups apple juice

2 cinnamon sticks

5 entire cloves

1/4 teaspoon ground nutmeg

1 cut of new ginger or 1/2 teaspoon vanilla concentrate (discretionary)

Juice of around 50% of an orange or lemon

Guidelines:

In a pan, combine the apple juice, cinnamon sticks, entire cloves, ground nutmeg, and new ginger or vanilla concentrate if utilized.

Crush the juice of around 50% of an orange or lemon into the combination.

Heat the blend over medium intensity until it starts to stew, staying away from a bubble.

Allow it to stew for 15-20 minutes for the flavors to implant.

Eliminate heat, strain the fluid to eliminate flavors, and serve warm.

This variety adds a fiery and reviving citrus component to the flavored fruity dessert mixture. Partake in your citrus-implanted creation!

Tropical Turmeric Infusion

Tropical Turmeric Imbuement is a tasty mix consolidating the glow of turmeric with tropical notes, making an invigorating and sweet-smelling refreshment.

This imbuement frequently incorporates fixings like turmeric, ginger, lemongrass, and maybe a touch of coconut or citrus for an even and calming tropical experience. It's known for its potential medical advantages and lively flavor profile.

The calming properties of turmeric, combined with the stomach-related advantages of ginger and the citrusy newness of lemongrass, make Tropical

Turmeric Imbuement delightful as well as possibly strong of generally speaking prosperity. It's usually appreciated both hot and chilled.

The energetic yellow tone of the mixture comes from curcumin, the dynamic compound in turmeric, known for its cancer-prevention agent properties. This mix offers a superb option in contrast to conventional teas, furnishing a lively and encouraging drink with a bit of colorful energy.

Preparing Tropical Turmeric Mixture includes soaking the mix in steaming hot water for a few minutes, permitting the flavors to merge. A few varieties could incorporate extra components like dark pepper to upgrade turmeric retention or a bit of honey for pleasantness. It's a flexible beverage, versatile to different inclinations.

Whether you're tasting it as a morning shot in the arm or slowing down at night, the Tropical Turmeric Implantation gives a tactile excursion, moving you to a tropical heaven with each taste. Trying different things with various soaking times and serving temperatures can additionally fit the experience you would prefer.

Past its captivating flavor, the imbuement's potential medical advantages have prompted its notoriety. Turmeric is accepted to have calming and cancer-prevention agent properties, while ginger adds to stomach-related prosperity. As you partake in this tropical mix, you're enjoying a wonderful beverage as well as possibly supporting your general well-being.

The mixture's sweet-smelling profile is an ensemble of warm heartiness from turmeric, a zingy kick from ginger, and a citrusy lift from lemongrass. This agreeable mix isn't simply a refreshment; a sensorial encounter draws in your taste buds and transports you to sun-kissed tropical scenes with each nuanced taste.

The particular fixings in a Tropical Turmeric Mixture can change, however normal parts include:

Turmeric: Adds warmth and an unmistakable brilliant variety.

Ginger: Contributes a fiery kick and possible stomach-related benefits.

Lemongrass: Implants a citrusy and natural note.

Coconut: Gives a rich and tropical hint in certain varieties.

Citrus Zing: Adds a brilliant and invigorating component.

Dark Pepper (discretionary): At times included to improve turmeric retention.

Honey or Sugar (discretionary): Added for pleasantness.

These fixings cooperate to make a tasty and possibly well-being steady drink.

Here is a straightforward recipe for Tropical Turmeric Implantation:

Fixings:

1 teaspoon ground turmeric or new turmeric cuts

1 teaspoon ground ginger

1 tail of lemongrass, hacked

1 teaspoon destroyed coconut (discretionary)

Zing of a portion of a lemon or lime

A spot of dark pepper (discretionary)

Honey or sugar to taste (discretionary)

Guidelines:

Bubble 2 cups of water in a pot.

Add turmeric, ginger, lemongrass, coconut (if utilizing), citrus zing, and dark pepper (if utilizing) to the bubbling water.

Lessen intensity and let it stew for around 5-7 minutes to permit the flavors to merge.

Strain the imbuement into cups.

Add honey or sugar to taste.

Partake in your Tropical Turmeric Implantation hot, or let it cool and serve over ice for a reviving chilled rendition.

Go ahead and change the fixing amounts because of your inclinations. Exploring different avenues regarding proportions can assist you with finding the ideal mix for your taste buds.

Here is a wind on the Tropical Turmeric Imbuement, making a Turmeric Citrus Cooler:

Fixings:

1 teaspoon ground turmeric or new turmeric cuts

1 teaspoon ground ginger

1 tablespoon lemongrass, finely slashed

1 teaspoon of destroyed coconut

Zing and juice of one orange

A spot of dark pepper

New mint leaves for decorating

Ice 3D shapes

Directions:

Bubble 2 cups of water in a pot.

Add turmeric, ginger, lemongrass, destroyed coconut, orange zing, and dark pepper to the bubbling water.

Permit it to stew for 5-7 minutes, guaranteeing the flavors merge.

Strain the imbuement into a pitcher and let it cool.

Once cooled, add the newly pressed squeezed orange.

Refrigerate the combination until chilled.

Serve over ice, decorated with new mint leaves.

This Turmeric Citrus Cooler offers a reviving and empowering turn on the customary implantation, ideal for a radiant day.

Portion Control and Timing

Controlling piece sizes and eating at ordinary spans can assist with keeping a decent eating regimen and backing in general well-being. It forestalls gorging and manages energy levels for the day.

Segment control includes directing how much food you devour to meet your nourishing necessities without indulging. Tips incorporate utilizing more modest plates, estimating segments, and being aware of serving sizes.

Timing-wise, go for the gold and snacks to support energy. Eating every 3-4 hours balances out glucose levels. Breakfast launches your digestion, and spreading protein admission for the day can help muscle fix. Make sure to remain hydrated and pay attention to your body's appetite prompts.

For people with diabetes, segment control, and timing are urgent for overseeing glucose levels. Here are a few custom-made tips:

Adjusted Feasts: Incorporate a blend of mind-boggling starches, lean proteins, and sound fats in every dinner to assist with balancing out glucose.

More modest, Successive Feasts: Eating more modest, even dinners for the day can forestall enormous spikes or drops in glucose.

Carb Observing: Be aware of carb consumption, zeroing in on entire grains, vegetables, and natural products. Convey them uniformly across feasts.

Standard Checking: Monitor glucose levels routinely to comprehend what various food varieties and bits mean for your levels.

Steady Timing: Hold back nothing and bite times every day to lay out a normal that supports glucose for the executives.

Here are extra tips for diabetes executives:

Fiber-rich Food varieties: Incorporate high-fiber food sources like entire grains, vegetables, and vegetables in your eating regimen. Fiber balances out glucose levels.

Protein Equilibrium: Consolidate lean proteins like poultry, fish, tofu, and vegetables to assist with controlling yearning and keeping up with bulk.

Solid Fats: Pick wellsprings of sound fats like avocados, nuts, and olive oil. These can assist with overseeing glucose and backing in general heart well-being.

Hydration: Remain very much hydrated with water. Limit sweet beverages, and be wary of liquor utilization, which can influence glucose levels.

Customary Activity: Take part in normal actual work, as it can further develop insulin awareness. Talk with your medical services group to foster a reasonable activity plan.

Keep in mind, that individual reactions to food can fluctuate, so working intimately with medical services experts will assist with fitting these basic rules to your particular necessities.

The following are a couple of additional tips for diabetes the board:

Careful Eating: Focus on yearning and totality signals. Eat gradually, appreciating each chomp, which can forestall gorging.

Dinner Arranging: Plan feasts to guarantee an even and diabetes-accommodating eating routine. This stays away from incautious food decisions.

Limit Handled Food varieties: Lessen admission of profoundly handled and sweet food varieties, as they can cause quick spikes in glucose levels.

Customary Glucose Checking: Save a reliable timetable for observing glucose levels to follow examples and make fundamental changes.

Stress The board: Practice pressure-decreasing procedures like profound breathing or contemplation, as stress can influence glucose levels.

Medicine Adherence: Accept endorsed meds as coordinated by your medical services supplier, and convey any worries or secondary effects speedily.

Keep in mind that customized exhortation from medical services experts is essential for overseeing diabetes successfully.

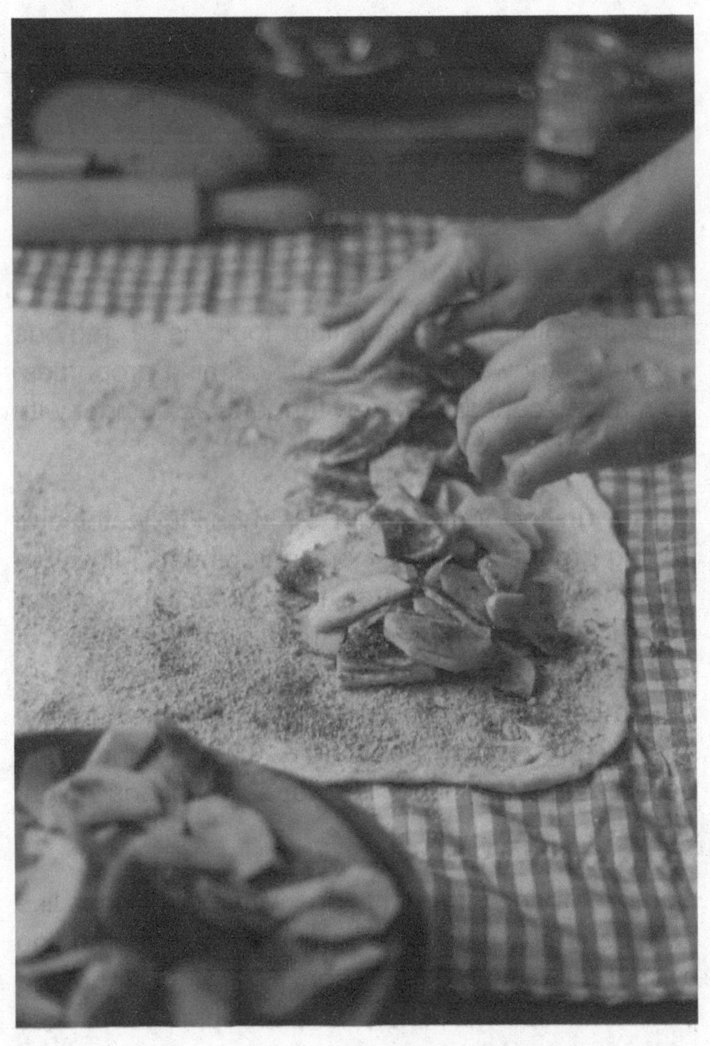

Chapter 5: Properties

Turmeric–Ginger Healing Tonic

Turmeric-Ginger recuperating tonic is a famous beverage known for its possible calming properties. To make it, consolidate new turmeric and ginger with water, and add honey or lemon for taste.

To set up the tonic, begin by bubbling water and adding ground or cut turmeric and ginger. Allow it to stew for around 10 minutes, then, at that point, strain the fluid. You can improve the flavor with a hint of honey and a crush of lemon. This tonic is remembered to help save well-being and give cancer prevention agents. Keep in mind, that balance is vital, and individual reactions might fluctuate.

Consider trying different things with extra fixings like dark pepper to upgrade turmeric ingestion or adding a spot of cinnamon for some zing. Change the pleasantness and sharpness as per your taste inclinations.

You can redo the turmeric-ginger tonic further by integrating spices like mint or basil for an invigorating turn. Certain individuals like to incorporate a hint of apple juice vinegar for added potential medical advantages.

Explore different avenues regarding varieties by mixing the tonic with green tea or a homegrown tea of your decision. This can present new flavors and extra medical advantages. Guarantee that the fixings utilized to line up with your inclinations and dietary requirements.

Here is a fundamental recipe for a turmeric-ginger mending tonic:

Fixings:

1-2 creeps of new turmeric root, ground or cut

1-2 creeps of new ginger root, ground or cut

4 cups of water

Honey, to taste (discretionary)

Lemon juice, to taste (discretionary)

Extra discretionary fixings: dark pepper, cinnamon, mint, basil, apple juice vinegar

Go ahead and change amounts given your inclinations and wanted flavor profile.

Here is a basic recipe for the Turmeric-Ginger Mending Tonic:

Fixings:

1-2 crawls of new turmeric root, ground or cut

1-2 crawls of new ginger root, ground or cut

4 cups of water

Discretionary: 1-2 tablespoons of honey (conform to taste)

Discretionary: New lemon juice (conform to taste)

Discretionary: Touch of dark pepper, cinnamon, or spices like mint/basil

Discretionary: 1-2 tablespoons of apple juice vinegar

Directions:

In a pot, heat 4 cups of water to the point of boiling.

Add the ground or cut turmeric and ginger to the bubbling water.

Diminish the intensity and let the combination stew for around 10 minutes.

Strain the fluid to eliminate the turmeric and ginger pieces.

Permit the fluid to cool somewhat before adding honey, lemon juice, and any discretionary elements for some extra zing.

Mix well and taste, changing pleasantness or sharpness depending on the situation.

Empty the tonic into a glass or store it in the fridge for a reviving, well-being-helping drink.

Make sure to talk with a medical services professional, particularly if you have explicit well-being concerns or are on drugs. Partake in your Turmeric-Ginger Recuperating Tonic!

Beetroot Carrot Immunity Booster

Beetroot and carrot are rich in cancer prevention agents and supplements that might uphold resistant well-being. Remembering them for your eating routine can add to a balanced way to deal with supporting invulnerability.

Both beetroot and carrots contain nutrients like An and C, fundamental for resistant capability. Moreover, they give minerals and phytonutrients that add to general prosperity. Consider integrating them into servings of mixed greens, squeezes, or cooked dishes for a scrumptious and nutritious lift.

Beetroot's nitrates might assist with further developing the bloodstream, while carrots offer beta-carotene, a forerunner to vitamin A. These supplements support different parts of well-being, including heart capability and vision. Counting various brilliant vegetables guarantees a different scope of resistance helping intensifies your eating routine.

Both beetroot and carrots contain fiber, advancing a solid stomach-related framework. The fiber content keeps up with stomach well-being, which is connected to generally speaking invulnerable capability. Make sure to appreciate them as a component of a fair eating regimen to expand their advantages.

Also, beetroot has mitigating properties, possibly supporting diminishing aggravation in the body. Carrots, with their cell reinforcements, add to battling oxidative pressure, which can influence insusceptible well-being decidedly. A brilliant plate with these vegetables upholds insusceptibility as well as by and large balanced nourishment.

Remembering beetroot and carrots for your eating routine can likewise give a characteristic wellspring of energy, because of their mix of sugars and supplements. Whether delighted in crude, cooked or squeezed, these vegetables offer a scrumptious method for improving your general imperativeness and backing your resistant framework.

Also, beetroot contains betalains, intensifies that have cancer prevention agents and calming properties. Carrots, known for their beta-carotene, support skin wellbeing, going about as a protection boundary against microbes. Joining these components makes a strong blend that adds to a vigorous insusceptible framework and general prosperity.

To make a beetroot-carrot insusceptibility supporter, you'll require:

Beetroot: Washed, stripped, and cleaved.

Carrots: Washed, stripped, and cut.

Discretionary: Ginger - for added flavor and likely calming benefits.

Lemon juice: Newly pressed for a citrusy kick and L-ascorbic acid.

Discretionary: Apple - for normal pleasantness and additional supplements.

Mix these fixings into a smooth squeeze or integrate them into servings of mixed greens or dishes in light of your inclination. Change amounts given your taste and want consistency.

Here is a straightforward recipe for a Beetroot-Carrot Insusceptibility Sponsor Juice:

Fixings:

1 medium-sized beetroot (washed, stripped, and slashed)

2-3 medium-sized carrots (washed, stripped, and cut)

1 little piece of ginger (discretionary, stripped)

1 tablespoon of new lemon juice

1 apple (discretionary, cored and cleaved)

Water or coconut water (depending on the situation for wanted consistency)

Directions:

Place beetroot, carrots, ginger, and apple (if utilizing) in a blender.

Add new lemon juice for a citrusy flavor.

Add water or coconut water to assist with mixing. Change the amount given your favored thickness.

Mix until smooth. Strain if you lean toward a smoother juice.

Fill a glass, and it's prepared to appreciate!

Go ahead and modify the recipe in light of your taste inclinations and dietary necessities.

Here is a scrumptious Beetroot-Carrot Salad recipe:

Fixings:

1 medium-sized beetroot (washed, stripped, and ground)

2-3 medium-sized carrots (washed, stripped, and ground)

1 tablespoon olive oil

1 tablespoon apple juice vinegar

Salt and pepper to taste

New spices (parsley, cilantro) for embellish (discretionary)

Directions:

In a blending bowl, consolidate ground beetroot and carrots.

In a little bowl, whisk together olive oil, apple juice vinegar, salt, and pepper to make the dressing.

Pour the dressing over the ground vegetables and throw until all around covered.

Permit the plate of mixed greens to marinate for a couple of moments to upgrade flavors.

Embellish with new spices whenever wanted.

Serve and partake in this energetic and nutritious Beetroot-Carrot Salad!

This salad isn't just delicious but additionally loaded with invulnerable helping supplements.

Pomegranate Cherry Vitality Splash

Pomegranate Cherry Imperativeness Sprinkle might help diabetes patients because of its cell reinforcements, nutrients, and potential glucose guideline properties tracked down in pomegranates. Nonetheless, it's fundamental to talk with a medical care proficient for customized guidance because of individual wellbeing needs.

Pomegranates contain cell reinforcements like anthocyanins and polyphenols, which might make mitigating impacts and add to general well-being. A few examinations propose that pomegranate utilization could assist with overseeing glucose levels and further develop insulin responsiveness. Cherries likewise have a lower glycemic file contrasted with many organic products, which might be useful for diabetes the board.

Also, the fiber content in the two pomegranates and cherries might assist with dialing back the retention of sugars, possibly adding to more readily glucose control. It's critical to take note that while these organic products can be important for a reasonable eating regimen for diabetes, observing piece sizes and generally sugar admission is fundamental.

Besides, the normal pleasantness of pomegranates and cherries can offer a delightful option in contrast to refined sugars, supporting overseeing desires. The elevated degrees of nutrients, for example, L-ascorbic acid, in these organic products may likewise uphold safe capability, a viewpoint critical for generally speaking wellbeing, especially for those with diabetes.

Besides, the likely calming properties of pomegranates and cherries could help diabetes patients, as constant aggravation is related to insulin opposition. The presence of specific mixtures, such as ellagic corrosive in pomegranates, may add to these calming impacts. Consolidating different supplement-rich food varieties, including pomegranates and cherries, into an even eating regimen can assume a positive part in overseeing diabetes, yet individual reactions might change.

Likewise, the polyphenols in pomegranates and cherries might have cardiovascular advantages, which is critical for diabetes patients as they are at a higher gamble of heart-related issues. These natural products might uphold heart well-being by further developing cholesterol levels and diminishing oxidative pressure. Notwithstanding, keeping an all-encompassing way to deal with diabetes on the board, including ordinary activity and predictable observing, is urgent.

Moreover, the presence of anthocyanins in cherries might add to their potential calming and cell reinforcement impacts, which could be valuable for overseeing diabetes-related entanglements. A few examinations recommend that anthocyanins may assist with further developing insulin responsiveness and decrease markers of irritation. Nonetheless, continuous examination is expected to comprehend the degree of these advantages completely.

For a Pomegranate Cherry Imperativeness Sprinkle, you should seriously mull over the accompanying fixings:

Pomegranate seeds or squeeze

New or frozen cherries

Water or shining water

Ice 3D shapes

Discretionary: a sprinkle of lemon or lime juice for added punch

Consolidate these fixings as you would prefer inclination, and partake in a reviving and possibly helpful drink.

Here is a straightforward recipe for a Pomegranate Cherry Imperativeness Sprinkle:

Fixings:

1 cup pomegranate seeds or 100 percent pomegranate juice

1/2 cup new or frozen cherries, pitted

1 cup water or shimmering water

Ice blocks

Discretionary: 1 tablespoon lemon or lime juice

Directions:

In the case of utilizing new cherries, pit them.

In a blender, consolidate pomegranate seeds or squeeze, cherries, water (or shining water), and ice shapes.

Mix until smooth.

Whenever wanted, add lemon or lime juice for an additional kick and mix once more.

Strain the blend if you favor a smoother drink, or leave it as is for added fiber.

Fill a glass, add more ice if necessary, and top with a couple of pomegranate seeds or cherries.

Partake in your Pomegranate Cherry Imperativeness Sprinkle! Change the fixings to suit your taste inclinations.

Here is an elective Pomegranate Cherry Smoothie recipe:

Fixings:

1 cup pomegranate juice (unsweetened)

1/2 cup new or frozen cherries, pitted

1/2 cup Greek yogurt (plain or vanilla)

1 banana, stripped

1 tablespoon chia seeds

Ice 3D shapes

Directions:

In a blender, consolidate pomegranate juice, cherries, Greek yogurt, banana, chia seeds, and a small bunch of ice shapes.

Mix until smooth and rich.

Change the consistency by adding more ice or fluid if necessary.

Fill a glass and partake in this nutritious Pomegranate Cherry Smoothie.

This smoothie is rich in cell reinforcements, fiber, and protein, making it a delectable and empowering choice. Go ahead and tweak the recipe given your inclinations.

Chapter 6: Juicing as Part of a Healthy Lifestyle

Exercise and Diabetes Management

Ordinary activity can assist with overseeing diabetes by further developing insulin awareness and glucose control. It's fundamental to counsel your medical care supplier for customized direction on the sort and power of activities reasonable for your condition.

Integrate a blend of oxygen-consuming activities, such as lively strolling and strength preparation into your everyday practice. Go for the gold 150 minutes of moderate-power practice each week. Screen glucose levels when exercising, and remain hydrated. Acclimations to prescription or insulin might be required, so keep your medical services group informed about your actual work routine.

Also, know about hypoglycemia (low glucose) side effects during and after working out. Convey an effective starch source, similar to glucose tablets, and wear a clinical ID. Consistency in your work-out daily practice and a decent eating regimen are key parts of successful diabetes executives. Ordinary check-ups with your medical care group will help adjust your methodology.

Consider taking part in exercises you appreciate to make practice a maintainable piece of your way of life. Screen how your body answers various activities and changes as needed. Weight the board is additionally pivotal for diabetes control, as losing abundant weight can decidedly influence insulin awareness. Continuously focus on security and talk with medical care experts for custom-fitted exhortation.

Integrate both oxygen-consuming activities, like strolling or cycling, and obstruction preparing, such as weightlifting, to accomplish far-reaching medical advantages. Watch out for feelings of anxiety, as stress can affect glucose levels. Predictable rest is imperative as well, as it impacts general prosperity and can influence glucose digestion. Take a stab at an all-encompassing way to deal with diabetes the executives that incorporate a way of life factors past activity alone.

Guarantee you check your glucose levels consistently and remain receptive to how your body answers different food varieties and exercises. Defining practical objectives and celebrating little accomplishments can assist with keeping up with inspiration. If you experience any progressions in your well-being or notice vacillations in glucose levels, speedily speak with your medical care group for acclimations to your diabetes the executives plan.

Remain aware of your carb consumption and select complex starches with a lower glycemic file. This can add to more readily glucose control. Hydration is fundamental; hydrate routinely, particularly when working out. Ultimately, consider joining support gatherings or networks to share encounters and gain extra bits of knowledge about overseeing diabetes through a cooperative methodology.

Hydration and Other Healthy Habits

For diabetes patients, remaining hydrated is pivotal to assist with managing glucose levels. Furthermore, keeping a reasonable eating routine, standard activity, and checking sugar admission is fundamental for overseeing diabetes.

Consolidating fiber-rich food varieties, similar to entire grains and vegetables, can support controlling glucose. Segment control and feast timing are significant, and it's valuable to pick food varieties with a low glycemic file. Standard observing of glucose levels stresses the executives, and satisfactory rest likewise adds to general diabetes

Counting lean proteins, for example, poultry or fish, in your feast can assist with settling glucose. Choose solid fats like avocados and nuts while restricting soaked and trans fats. Normal active work, such as lively strolling, upholds insulin responsiveness. It's fundamental to keep away from sweet drinks and focus on water or homegrown teas. Keep in mind, that individual requirements change, so working intimately with your medical services group guarantees a balanced diabetes-the-board plan.

Routinely checking blood glucose levels and keeping a record can give experiences as examples and assist with changing way-of-life decisions as needed. Building an emotionally supportive network, including loved ones, can offer close-to-home help with overseeing diabetes. Instructing oneself about the condition cultivates better taking care of oneself.

Taking part in pressure-lessening exercises, like reflection or profound breathing activities, upholds generally speaking prosperity and can decidedly affect glucose levels. Ordinary eye tests and foot care are pivotal parts of diabetes the executives to early catch and address expected complexities. At long last, remaining informed about progressions in diabetes care and treatment choices considers informed decision-production with your medical services group.

Integrating standard high-impact workouts, such as strolling or cycling, further develops insulin awareness and generally cardiovascular well-being. Observing circulatory strain and cholesterol levels is significant for far-reaching diabetes care. Customary dental check-ups add to general well-being, as people with diabetes might be at a higher gamble of gum sickness. Consistency in solid propensities is key for long-haul prosperity.

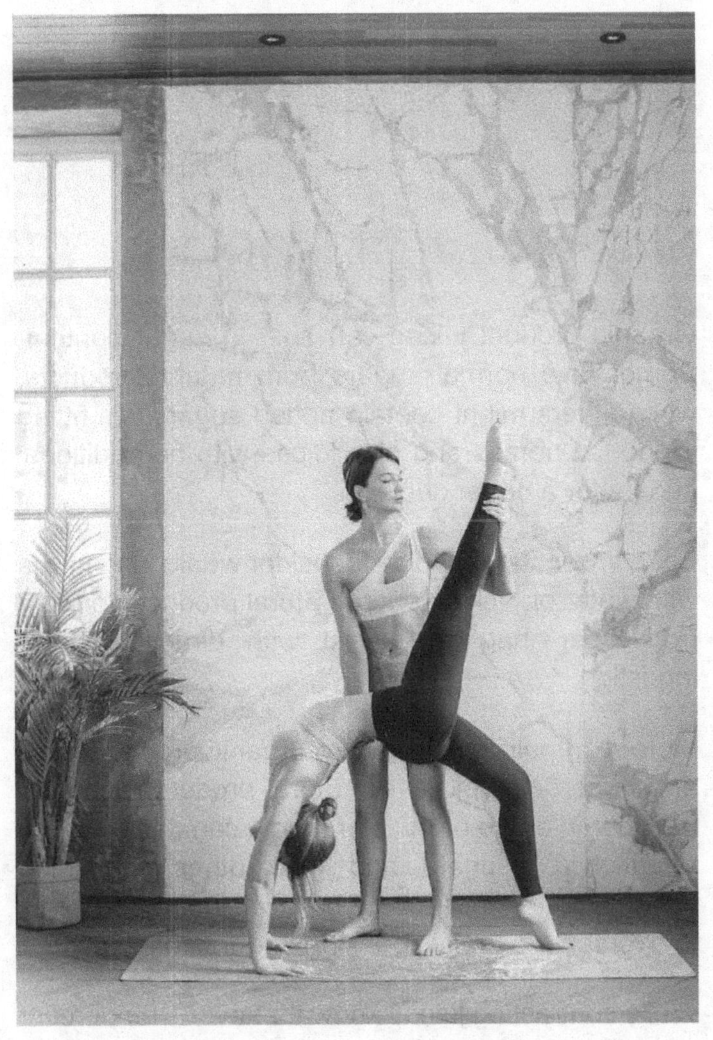

Chapter 7: Addressing Common Concerns

Sugar Content in Juices

Organic product juices can shift in sugar content. Some have normal sugars from natural products, while others might contain added sugars. It's fitting to look at names and pick juices with no additional sugars for a better decision.

For a lower sugar choice, consider weakening juices with water or picking entire natural products to profit from fiber that can assist with directing sugar ingestion.

Moreover, polishing off entire organic products is by and large desirable over natural product juices, as the fiber in entire organic products can dial back the retention of sugars and give other nourishing advantages. Continuously be aware of piece sizes to oversee generally speaking sugar consumption.

While contrasting juices know that even 100 percent organic product juices can be high in normal sugars. Deciding on new, natively constructed squeezes or picking entire natural products over juices can add to a more adjusted and nutritious eating regimen. It's vital to figure out some kind of harmony and be aware of your general sugar utilization for better well-being.

Consider integrating various natural products into your eating routine to profit from various supplements. While certain organic products are normally better, others offer a more tart or tart taste. This variety can improve your general healthful admission and give a fantastic scope of flavors without depending exclusively on sweet choices.

Assuming you mean to decrease sugar consumption, you could investigate choices like imbued water with cuts of citrus, berries, or spices. Along these lines, you can partake in a reviving drink with negligible or no additional sugars. Remaining hydrated with water is an amazing decision for general well-being.

Recall that control is vital. In any event, while picking lower-sugar choices, being aware of part estimates keeps a fair eating routine. Remaining informed about nourishing substances and settling on cognizant decisions lines up with a better way of life.

Interactions with Medications

Certain prescriptions, similar to beta-blockers or thiazide diuretics, can impact glucose levels and cover the side effects of hypoglycemia. Liquor utilization ought to be moderate and joined by food to forestall unforeseen glucose changes. It's imperative to keep a complete rundown of all drugs, enhancements, and way of life factors for your medical care supplier to settle on informed conclusions about your diabetes therapy plan. Normal check-ups and correspondence are critical for ideal diabetes care.

Make sure to screen for indications of hypoglycemia, like wooziness or disarray, particularly while presenting new meds. A few prescriptions might require changes in your diabetes the executives plan. Homegrown enhancements can likewise be associated with diabetes prescriptions, so illuminate your medical services supplier about any elective treatments you're thinking about.

Furthermore, be mindful of expected connections with non-professionally prescribed drugs like painkillers or cold prescriptions, as they can affect glucose levels. Consistently survey your blood glucose readings and offer them to your medical care supplier to evaluate the adequacy of your ongoing drug routine. Any progressions in your well-being or way of life ought to be conveyed speedily to guarantee a proactive way to deal with overseeing diabetes and forestalling difficulties.

Besides, a few prescriptions, similar to specific statins, could have a double advantage by both overseeing cholesterol levels and giving cardiovascular security to people with diabetes. Notwithstanding, talking about the likely advantages and dangers of every prescription with your medical services provider is pivotal. Keeping a cooperative and informed relationship with your medical services group is fundamental for exploring the intricacies of diabetes with the executives and streamlining your general well-being.

It's vital to know about expected cooperation between diabetes meds and different circumstances you might have. For instance, kidney or liver issues can affect how your body processes prescriptions. Consistently survey your clinical history with your medical care supplier to guarantee that your diabetes executives line up with your general well-being.

Furthermore, way-of-life factors like changes in diet, workout schedules, or feelings of anxiety can impact how your body answers diabetes drugs. Keeping your medical services supplier informed about such changes takes into account acclimations to your therapy plan on a case-by-case basis. Take a stab at open correspondence, stick to endorsed prescription regimens, and go to normal check-ups to guarantee your diabetes the board stays compelling and customized to your developing well-being needs.

In specific circumstances, prescriptions utilized for diabetes executives might cause secondary effects.

It's critical to report any strange side effects or unfriendly responses to your medical services supplier speedily. Routinely booked arrangements give you a chance to examine any worries, survey your general well-being, and make essential changes per your diabetes treatment plan for ideal outcomes. Keep in mind that your dynamic contribution to your medical care is vital to effective diabetes executives.

Success Stories and Testimonials

Individuals have made progress in overseeing diabetes by taking on a low-starch diet, rehearsing segment control, and consolidating customary actual work. Furthermore, support from medical care groups, diabetes teachers, and online networks plays had an urgent impact in enabling people to explore their excursion.

A few people have shared tales about critical upgrades in their diabetes the executives by zeroing in on pressure decrease methods, satisfactory rest, and keeping a predictable everyday practice. Customized approaches, like tracking down the right harmony between drugs and grasping individual triggers, have additionally added to positive results.

It's motivating to see the assorted ways individuals take to make progress in overseeing diabetes.

Others have revealed accomplishment with persistent glucose observing frameworks, which give ongoing experiences into glucose levels, considering more exact acclimations to slim down and prescription. Investigating elective treatments, similar to care practices and needle therapy, has been embraced by some as reciprocal systems in their diabetes executives. These accounts feature the significance of customized approaches and the ability to investigate different instruments and strategies.

Certain people have made progress in overseeing diabetes by embracing innovation, for example, cell phone applications that assist with following feasts, screening active work, and giving suggestions for drugs. Associating with a steady local area, either face to face or on the web has demonstrated gainful for some, cultivating a feeling of support and shared encounters. These different methodologies highlight the significance of fitting procedures to individual requirements and inclinations in the excursion to oversee diabetes effectively.

Also, examples of overcoming adversity frequently stress the meaning of ordinary check-ups and open correspondence with medical care experts. Working together with a medical care group to define sensible objectives and consistently reevaluate the administration plan assists people with remaining focused and making fundamental changes. A unique interaction includes continuous learning, variation, and the obligation to a comprehensive way to deal with well-being.

Frequently Asked Questions

What is diabetes?

Diabetes is an ongoing condition where the body battles to control glucose levels successfully.

What are the fundamental kinds of diabetes?

The primary kinds are Type 1 and Type 2 diabetes. Type 1 is an immune system condition, while Type 2 is frequently connected to way of life factors.

How is diabetes analyzed?

Diabetes is normally analyzed through blood tests estimating glucose levels.

What are the normal side effects of diabetes?

Successive peeing, over-the-top thirst, unexplained weight reduction, and exhaustion are normal side effects.

How could diabetes be made due?

The executives include way of life changes, drugs, insulin treatment, and standard checking of glucose levels.

What is HbA1c, and for what reason is it significant?

HbA1c is a blood test that reflects normal glucose levels for more than a while, giving a drawn-out perspective on glycemic control.

What dietary rules should diabetics observe?

A fair eating regimen with controlled starch consumption, zeroing in on entire food sources, is vital. Discussion with a dietitian is frequently suggested.

How truly does practice influence diabetes?

Customary actual work assists control of blood sugar levels, further develops insulin awareness, and supports generally speaking wellbeing.

Might diabetes at any point be forestalled?

A solid way of life decisions, for example, keeping a fair eating routine, remaining truly dynamic, and overseeing pressure, can lessen the gamble of creating Type 2 diabetes.

What would it be a good idea for me to do in the event of a hypoglycemic (low glucose) episode?

Polish off an effective wellspring of glucose, like natural product juice or glucose tablets. Continuously convey a wellspring of effective sugar.

What are the possible inconveniences of diabetes?

Confusions might incorporate coronary illness, kidney harm, nerve harm, and eye issues. Normal check-ups help recognize and deal with these issues early.

How frequently would it be advisable for me to check my glucose levels?

Recurrence fluctuates, however, it's generally expected to look at levels on various occasions every day, particularly around dinners and before sleep time.

Is it ok for diabetics to polish off liquor?

Control is critical. Talk with your medical care supplier to comprehend what liquor might mean for your particular circumstance.

Will pressure affect glucose levels?

Indeed, stress can raise glucose levels. Stress-the-board methods, similar to contemplation or exercise, can be helpful.

Which job does prescription play in diabetes the board?

Prescription, including oral medications and insulin infusions, might be recommended to assist with controlling glucose levels. The sort and dose rely upon individual necessities.

Is it feasible for diabetes to go into abatement?

For some purposes, way of life changes and weight reduction might prompt abatement, particularly in Type 2 diabetes. Be that as it may, it is pivotal to continuous checking.

What's the association between diabetes and foot care?

Diabetes can influence flow and nerve capability in the feet. Standard foot assessments and appropriate consideration assist with forestalling confusion.

Might pregnancy at any point influence diabetes on the board?

Pregnancy can influence glucose levels, requiring close observation and now and then acclimations to treatment plans.

Are there care groups for individuals with diabetes?

Indeed, numerous networks offer care groups where people with diabetes can share encounters and counsel.

How does smoking influence diabetes?

Smoking expands the gamble of intricacies related to diabetes, like cardiovascular sickness. It is unequivocally encouraged to Stop smoking.

Continuously talk with medical care experts for customized counsel in light of your particular ailments and necessities.